MAMA BARE
THE GRIZZLY TRUTHS OF MOTHERHOOD

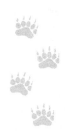

Nicole Obenshine

Praeclarus Press, LLC
©2021 Nicole Obenshine. All rights reserved.

www.PraeclarusPress.com

Praeclarus Press, LLC
2504 Sweetgum Lane
Amarillo, Texas 79124 USA
806-367-9950
www.PraeclarusPress.com

DISCLAIMER

The information contained in this publication is advisory only and is not intended to replace sound clinical judgment or individualized patient care. The author disclaims all warranties, whether expressed or implied, including any warranty as the quality, accuracy, safety, or suitability of this information for any particular purpose.

ISBN: 978-1-946665-49-2

Cover Design: Ken Tackett
Developmental Editing: Kathleen Kendall-Tackett
Copyediting: Chris Tackett
Layout & Design: Nelly Murariu

Dedications

I want to dedicate this book to my two boys, for without them, there would be no words to fill these pages. I want to also thank my husband for helping create these beautiful souls.

Dylan taught me how to be a Mother. He showed me that I was capable of getting through darkness and has inspired me to shine my light. He has created more joy in my heart than I ever thought was possible. He has challenged me to be better. I am forever grateful that his sweet soul chose our family and helped evolve me into my best self.

I want him to be proud of his Mama and know that he had a big impact on any success that I may meet.

Owyn taught me just how powerful and unstoppable I am. When I put my mind to something, there is truly nothing that can get in my way. He somehow has created even more joy than I ever thought was possible, especially the way he and Dylan love each other. He has proven me right in so many ways, and I am forever grateful for his sweet soul that chose our family at the most perfect time.

I want him to be proud of his Mama and know he had a big impact on any success that I may meet.

John, my husband, has been my rock and my support system throughout it all. He enables me to step into my authentic power and do what is best for our family. He may not always understand my madness, but he trusts that I have the best intentions for the safety and wellbeing of us all. Thank you for being by my side each and every day.

Lastly, for any future soul that may be guided into our family, I look forward to meeting you and seeing how you add to this story and contribute to the world's light the way Dylan and Owyn have. This is something only the Universe knows, and I will honor and trust that with sunrise faith.

I love you all so much.

To All the Mamas and Mamas to Be

You are doing the best you can. You are enough, and you are certainly not alone. No matter the road you travel, we all have one commonality, one fundamental quality that cannot be ignored; We create life. We are powerful beyond any measure of conscious logic. As a collective, we are unstoppable.

Mamas, you inspire me every day. You show me strength I never knew. You show me pure beauty, unconditional love, and foundations for living in your truth.

You deserve to know that you are magnificently worth all the goodness in this world. Your babies believe it, and you should too.

My hope for this book is to inspire those who feel defeated, stuck, or unworthy. I hope to give you a glimpse into how Motherhood really is and not just chalk it up to the highlight reel we have come to know.

I respect every Mother's journey and choice for their families, and honor, love, and support them without judgment. I will also ask you for the same in return as I unapologetically share mine.

Remember, you are your own best advocate; follow your gut, your heart, and your intuition.

You were born for this.

Thank you, I love you, you are enough, and certainly not alone.

Contents

Introduction

Hello, Beautiful Creators!

My name is Nicole. I most commonly identify as a Mother of two, a wife, and a healer. I am thrilled that you have picked up this book, physically or digitally, because I feel that every Mama should have a chance to tell their story, be empowered, and felt heard.

I have learned various "truths" about conception, pregnancy, and postpartum in the last few years and I want to fearlessly share my journey of Motherhood.

This book is a collection of stories of my struggles, my celebrations, my darkness, and my light, in my experiences, as well as those of other Moms, in hopes that *you* can feel less alone while reading.

I will fully admit that this book does not hold back; it does not sugarcoat reality. For example, you will soon know that I experienced what I called "Cottage Cheese Discharge" for the first 8 weeks of my first pregnancy while I was prescribed Progesterone to ensure that I was able to keep the baby. My loving husband had to assist in putting on my underwear for a solid month prior to giving birth both times, and I had daily horrendous visions of myself hanging from a ceiling fan in my Mom's kitchen as I battled PPOCD.

This is what actual Moms are going through each day, and it needs to become normal conversation.

Although this book is composed of my personal experiences, I know each path differs greatly from preconception to postpartum. I want to make sure that you know I honor each journey as uniquely beautiful or difficult. My hope is that this will give you hope, guidance, and relatability. Motherhood is not meant to be experienced alone. Let this book be part of your community.

When the idea for this book began, I had only experienced one perinatal journey, and days before speaking to the publisher, I found out that I was *unexpectedly* expecting baby number two. I am so excited about the timing because this journey has been vastly different from the first. I am writing this as I sit patiently waiting for baby O to arrive in a few short days/weeks. The perspective I now have can more deeply relate to an even wider audience, and I hope that I am able to give courage, comfort, or confidence to more Mothers who are in need.

Let's explore the truths that I have found over the last 5 years.

Enjoy!

Love & Gratitude,

Nicole

Truth 1 | YOU ARE NEVER READY

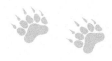
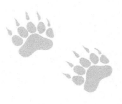

Yes, you can have the job, house, husband, or wife. Yes, you can be fertile and filled with baby fever. However, you will never be 100% ready for what a baby brings to your world. Even throughout pregnancy, you can be totally confident of what you will be doing when the baby gets here, but things will not be like you thought. And that's *okay*! That is part of the journey of life. It is unknown to anyone; your Mother doesn't know, and your doctor doesn't know. Only that little miracle knows. There is a quote that you can be a perfect Mom until you have kids. You can decide that you will breastfeed, never co-sleep, and personally make fully organic baby food, then your baby is colic, you are tired, and it's way too easy to just buy the little pouch of apples. And that's *okay*!

I want any woman thinking about having children that you are as ready as you can be because you were born for this. The generational and societal expectations are not realistic. All you have to know is how to love that bundle of joy. That will guide you toward all the "right" decisions for your family.

I never wanted children, solely because I could not fathom the idea of being able to carry and birth a child with how much fear I had around anything medical. Then I met my husband and things changed. I was still scared, but it was a thought that crossed my mind occasionally. I had stipulations, though. We needed to have a home of our own. We needed to have $10K in the bank. We had to both have secure full-time jobs. I had to lose weight. We had to figure it all out beforehand. Most of those boxes were checked when we started to try, but what I learned is that none of them mattered.

My first son, Dylan, was "very planned," as you can see. Even when we did start trying, it took 12 months of a bad guessing game and 2 IUI cycles to conceive. That should have been my first sign that this was not up to me. My second son, Owyn, came like a whirlwind once we started "discussing" having baby number two. You would have thought that I learned my lesson with the first, but no, trying to plan the "perfect" time to expand the family blew up in our faces when we unexpectedly got pregnant without any fertility help about a year earlier than we were discussing. We had no money in the bank. We had bigger bills. My husband left his secure job for one with half the income. And I had been at my heaviest weight. Oh, and to top it off, we had just decided to host a teenage exchange student from August to June who would be occupying our third bedroom.

But guess what? He is here, he is healthy and happy, and I am too. We were not ready for Owyn, but I am the happiest I have ever been with these two beautiful boys. The bills are getting paid, and even in a pandemic, this has been an amazing journey.

So, take this in stride. You can become a Mother without being ready and you will be a damn good one.

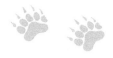

Truth 2 | CONCEPTION LOOKS DIFFERENT FOR EVERYONE

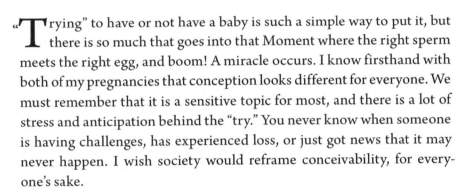

"Trying" to have or not have a baby is such a simple way to put it, but there is so much that goes into that Moment where the right sperm meets the right egg, and boom! A miracle occurs. I know firsthand with both of my pregnancies that conception looks different for everyone. We must remember that it is a sensitive topic for most, and there is a lot of stress and anticipation behind the "try." You never know when someone is having challenges, has experienced loss, or just got news that it may never happen. I wish society would reframe conceivability, for everyone's sake.

When I was "ready" to try for Dylan, it was a bad guessing game that we played for a year. Negative test after negative test. I bought the bulk test strips from Amazon, and you bet I went through every one of them during this time. We finally made the decision to see a reproductive endocrinologist.

Disclaimer: I will talk about the Universe a lot throughout this book. You can interchange that word with your personal deity that you reference (God, Angels, Source, Jesus, etc.). I am referring to the higher consciousness that is present in all our lives.

The Universe was on our side when scheduling the appointment. I had been tracking my cycles, and I made the appointment with my logical mind to not be on my period, thinking that it was like when you go to the gynecologist. Well, that was the first sign that I had no control over this process because my cycle came late, and it was smack right in the middle when we went for our consultation. Little did I know, it was a good thing, and we were able to start Medication Cycle #1 *that day.*

This journey started quicker than I anticipated. It was a lot of blood-work and ultrasounds over the next few weeks, and a dreaded two week wait. That cycle was unsuccessful. However, I learned so much about my body, the process, and what I had to shift for this to work.

The second cycle began, and I always had fertility crystals in my bra. I did fertility meditations, and I practiced detachment. I was putting my faith in the Universe. One thing I learned from cycle one was that when I received the trigger shot, it consisted of the pregnancy hormone. That being said, if I were to take a test, it would be positive. I had never seen a positive test result before, so I took one and felt how I believed I would feel when it was a true test. I relished in that feeling and surrendered to the rest of the process. I did a lot of self-Reiki and more meditation to keep my mind relaxed and detached during the two-week wait.

Then the other side of the spectrum happened. My sister, who was not trying to have a baby, called to let me know that she was unexpected-ly pregnant on the same day I started spotting and took a negative test for Cycle #2. My concern shifted from my negative result to her positive one because conception can be hard when it happens easily too. She had obsta-cles to figure out and reactions to prepare for. It was no longer about me. I am convinced that the Universe aligned these events on purpose because two days later, when I went to start Cycle #3 at the doctors, the bloodwork came back positive.

That's right, my sister and I were due two weeks apart to the day. Our pregnancies, like our conception, looked very different, but we had two beautiful babies three weeks apart to the day. So, if these scenarios can be so different for two women who came from the same womb, imagine how different every single one of our experiences can be. Remember that next time you ask a friend when they plan to have a baby or even another baby. Sometimes fertility challenges come after the first baby. It can get even more intrinsically different.

With my second pregnancy, we proactively saw the fertility doctor to answer some questions we had about medication, birth control, and protocol for baby #2. In my mind, it was about a year away from trying, and we wanted to leave time for anything that may have needed to be done (weaning off medication/trying on our own before we did treatment again). His recommendation was to see how my cycles were since having Dylan.

So, the plan was for three months to track them and get back on birth control until we were ready. I had my first 28-day cycle ever. I was excited, but then I had a 40 day one, so it was not a long-lasting excitement. I was waiting for my next period to start back on birth control, and I had started spotting on a Sunday. I was trying the new "Flex" ring that someone had recommended to me, so I used that for Monday, and then noticed it never fully came on, and by Wednesday night, left altogether. This had been a familiar occurrence when I was pregnant with Dylan. So, Thursday morning, I woke up, and in my gut, I knew I was pregnant. Later that night, I took a test, and sure enough, it was positive.

In my experiences alone, there have been so many variations of conception. Expand that to family and friends, acquaintances, and strangers; the possibilities are endless. We need to understand this so we can be aware of the words we say when couples get married, or if someone has a child outside of marriage. We need to know that no matter how it happens, it is a miracle. We need to know that women (and men) can have many insecurities around fertility, loss, and sterility. So be kind, be cognitive, and when in doubt, be silent.

For you Mamas who are trying right now, I see you. The best advice I can give is to remain hopeful, trust in your body, feel the feelings of a positive test, and surrender to the Universe. You are a Creator.

On a fertility note, if you must go through treatment, or if you have experienced loss, have your progesterone levels checked. If you need to supplement, please do yourself a favor and ask for the oral version. The alternative is a suppository that basically gives you discharge that could only be described as cottage cheese. You are going through enough in early pregnancy; you don't need that crap. With Dylan, I did not know any better; it was a fun time. With Owyn, it was just another vitamin to take.

Try This One! See It to Conceive It.

Like I had mentioned in Truth #2, I had taken a test after my trigger shot, knowing it would be a false positive. Why would I do such a thing? Because of the power of visualization and manifestation. When we can see something clear in our minds and decide it is ours, it appears in our reality. If you are not currently in fertility treatments, there are other ways to elicit this result. Emotions are even more powerful than thoughts, and your subconscious mind cannot reject what it is told. Therefore, if you believe you are seeing a positive test, create that image in your mind and feel all the emotions you would when you do see those double lines.

You can absolutely put yourself into the frequency needed to conceive. If you do this, and then practice the Law of Detachment by not stressing and obsessing over the result. I promise that you will be closer to that beautiful miracle. Go to Mamabarebook.com for a list of fertility crystals, rituals, and an opportunity to schedule a complimentary Womb Light Healing if you have been trying to conceive for 12 months or longer.

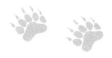

Truth 3 | PREGNANCY IS NOT ONE-SIZE-FITS-ALL

I can say the same thing about conception, Motherhood, and basic human existence in general. However, this truth is about gestation. There are a buttload of symptoms, complications, and overall issues that can happen during those 40(ish) weeks. As soon as you announce that you are expecting, the entire world has an opinion based on their own experience and wants to solicit all of their advice. Plus, they feel compelled to tell you horror stories that they have had or heard by others. Why does everyone think this is helpful? It isn't. You are already feeling emotions that you probably never have felt before. Your body is creating surges of chemicals and hormones that it never has before, and every woman in your life thinks it's beneficial to make your head spin even more.

Let's take a step back. I know you are already going to be Googling every little thing about the size of the baby, the foods you should and should not eat, and all the do's and don'ts outlined by WebMD and the mainstream medical community. So, if you must, sure, go ahead. But make sure you read with an open mind and know it is not "law." I invite you to kindly tell anyone who tries to give you advice without you asking for it that you appreciate that they want to help but you have decided to take it day by day and see how your own experience plays out.

My experiences with both sons were completely different from each other. Also, if you remember, my sister and I were pregnant with our firsts at the exact same time (give or take 21 days), and we had completely different experiences, from the gender of the babies we carried to the ways we delivered.

You must think of pregnancy like a nursing bra. Some women will need bigger cup sizes, others bigger circumference, some like pretty ones, others solely for function, some will go completely bra-free, and others will always need one on to feel supported.

Because this book is about my journeys, I do want to express some important things that arose in mine. First, I never thought vomiting could be so "elegant." I mean that during my pregnancy with Dylan, I had morning sickness for about 5 weeks, and as a full-time employee, I spent a lot of this time at my office. Before conceiving, I perceived morning sickness to feel exactly like when you have a stomach bug or food poisoning. However, it is not. You feel like you must throw up, proceed to the bathroom, do your thing, and feel completely fine afterward until your next episode arises. So, there's a positive on a pretty sucky system. Another thing I want to touch on is my pregnancy with Owyn. I had this super awful pain and weakness arise in my pelvic area. It was the way my ligaments were stretching, and things were expanding. I was, luckily, introduced to the concept of Pelvic Floor Therapy and knew of a fantastic therapist. So, my advice is to all expecting Mamas. Find a local pelvic floor therapist. It's a gamechanger. None of these little helpful hints came to me by chance. I immersed myself in resources, information, and intentional communities in order to better help the Moms I knew who deserved to be informed.

Lastly, I am going to dive deep into pregnancy weight in the next truth. However, there is a different message I am trying to get across, so I want to touch on this here. Nutrition and exercise look different for every pregnancy. Cravings will happen; honor them. You may be a gym rat but are so incredibly tired you cannot fathom even tying your sneakers. Honor that. You are creating a human in your body. I promise that you will be okay. Give yourself grace here. Please do not beat yourself up over these two components during these 40 weeks. They will look different than your "normal" life.

Grace is a crucial practice that will be referenced a lot in these pages. It is so important to halt self-judgment and self-depreciation as quickly as you can. We are so conditioned to see the worst-case scenario, all the flaws, and the full negativity bias we are ingrained with, thanks to the ego. No matter your situation, know that it is just right for you. You are on this journey, so don't compare it to anyone else's. Every perinatal stage is not one-size-fits-all, especially pregnancy.

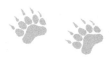

Truth 4 | THERE IS NO "RIGHT SIZE" FOR PREGNANCY

As a society, we are not great at understanding healthy vs. skinny. You can be healthy and overweight, and you can have the "perfect body" but not be healthy. Unfortunately, doctors also do not understand this concept. First, let me say, I understand the "factual" risks and complications that *could* occur due to higher BMIs in pregnancy, and like the last truth, this is not one size fits all. All I am saying is that we need to do a better job of looking at the individual and not the numbers.

Case in point; I was 260 lbs. when I got pregnant with Owyn. At almost every doctor's appointment, I was reminded of that, and not because I got on a scale. For both of my pregnancies, I had only gained about 20 lbs. Let's do some math. I had an average 8 lb. baby inside me, plus high fluid both times and a placenta. I'd say MOST if not all that weight was from the tiny human and life-sustaining system that my "overweight" body created. However, I was fat-shamed during my first pregnancy by a doctor, saying "you need to lose 100 lbs. You *should* only gain 10 lbs. during this entire pregnancy" and my fertility doctor saying, "you should start losing weight with your next meal" when we went to consult about baby #2.

Words can hurt, of course, but it went further than that. There were diagnoses, biases, and actions taken due to these beliefs, and that is what needs to change. So, Mama, if you are reading this right now at whatever size you are, know that you are not perfect, but you do not have to be in order to be the best Mother, the most powerful warrior, and the greatest human being on this planet.

Do not let our society knock you down during this time that you are creating life within your beautiful body. Yes, there will be stretch marks, flabby skin, and extra pounds all associated with the process, but those are the souvenirs that will remind you how freaking amazing you are. We also need to stop the "bounce back after baby" ploy and reframe it. We will never go backwards due to what we just endured, physically, emotionally and spiritually. We are Evolved. So getting to the new "best version" of yourself as a Mother is the Evolution. Looking forward and never bouncing back.

Weeks after both of my boys, I was back to "pre-pregnancy weight" without trying, which validated how many of those pounds were necessary for me to have. Even if that is not the case, it's *okay*.

I had two vaginal births: one in a hospital with an epidural and one in a birth center, unmedicated and unattached to monitors and IVs. No complications, no issues. Just my powerful 250 lb. body doing what it was *made* to do. Again, these are my experiences and my perceptions, but how many of you know someone who was overweight and had a vaginal delivery? What about a C-section? Okay, now how many of you know a "fit and thin" Mother who had a vaginal delivery? What about a C-Section?

My point is, there is no *one* way that this miracle happens for anyone, regardless of their size. So, can we stop acting like every overweight Mom must end in surgery because they will have some sort of complication? I am talking to you, OB/GYNs! And Mamas, I am also talking to you because if you feel like you are being "profiled," do not let it define your pregnancy, and advocate for yourself. I will go into more detail with this in the next Truth.

If you are reading this and you are thinking about conceiving or are in early pregnancy, know that your weight does not define your journey. If you are a Mama who hasn't lost every prego-pound yet, give yourself grace. You are beautiful. This is not a rollercoaster at an amusement park. The pregnancy ride does not have a "size" requirement.

As I am writing this, there is a movement going on in our country. A fight for equality and to stop systemic oppression due to the color of skin. I want to take some space to say that the maternal statistics for black women are devastating, and my hope is that this movement helps discover ways to fix this for good. All Moms deserve to feel empowered and radiant during pregnancy and birth. Feeling *safe* should not even be a thought, but for them, it is, and even though I cannot relate, I stand for change so that they can feel secure in their power as well—black Mothers matter. I will say it again, Black. Mothers. Matter. As a collective, if we advocate for ourselves, it unconsciously gives others the permission to advocate for themselves and begin to change the narrative around pregnancy, birth, Motherhood, and the care and support every single Mother deserves.

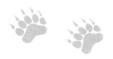
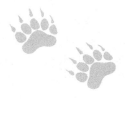

Truth 5 | You Know Best. Trust Yourself.

We are all in our own bodies *all* the time. We know ourselves best. As women, we have such beautiful divine feminine energy within us that allows us to intuitively "feel and know" things that the logical mind may not be able to conceive. Stay true to those feelings, Mama. They will be your best GPS on this journey from conception to postpartum and years beyond. Right now, pause and give yourself permission to receive all the messages you need to and give yourself permission to listen to them. They say the gut is the second brain, and we all know the expression "trust your gut." There is a reason.

During my first pregnancy, it was smooth sailing: normal office visits, normal symptoms. I didn't know too much about how intuitive I could be until 37 weeks when my water "broke." I quote that because, apparently, to doctors, it was just a high leak, and I was in false labor. That there's no way would I be having this baby that week. It was a Sunday afternoon. By Tuesday night, guess what I was holding in my arms? A beautiful baby boy. I was sent home from the hospital two times because it was "false labor." Back labor, nonetheless.

I had the stink about me for a couple of years about how I was so mad that I wasn't admitted. Knowing better now, I am happy that I did not get admitted until I was progressing more because there would have been induction pressure that probably would have led to surgery. My doula allowed me to honor my version until she finally reframed it. However, my wish is that I was just heard and validated. The doctors could have said, "Nicole, although you are experiencing these contractions and loss of fluid, it may be a couple of days until the next stage of labor starts. Go home and stay comfortable, and I will follow up with you at X time." Instead, I got, "you are only 37 weeks; we can't induce you, and you are not dilated. It's just false labor." So, what did I do? I was stuck in the pain and I was stuck in the anxiety of this pain lasting weeks. Luckily, I proved them wrong, and he was here within 48 hours, no Pitocin needed. But it's just another thing wrong with our system.

My second pregnancy took my self-advocacy to a whole other level. This entire pregnancy can only be described as "intuitive" from the day we found out we were expecting. I just woke up that morning (August 8, 2019) and knew it. I went to work as normal, and around 11 am, the nudging feeling I had got stronger, and I texted my husband, called my doctor, and sure enough, I was right. I also readjusted my due date from 4/16 to 4/4, and my contractions started at 2 am on what day? Saturday, April 4, 2020. Before we jump to the end, the juicy parts are all in the middle of this pregnancy.

I started out at my fertility doctor, on a progesterone supplement like my first, then moved to the OB/GYN Practice in the same office building as him. They delivered at the hospital that I had Dylan in, and they had a group of midwives, and I wanted a different experience this time around now that I was more confident in my ability to actually birth a human.

At my 15-week visit, I had an unusually high blood pressure reading. It was 155/110. Now, I know that is scary high, and I do not disagree with the doctors' concerns. It was how they handled the whole thing that did not sit well with me. First, I had never had a machine pump as slow as this one did. Second, they gave me a Glucose drink to go home with and drink before the next office visit, which was in one week. Third, they didn't give me a chance to monitor it for a day or two before throwing me on a pretty significant dose of medication. So, I went home and did some Googling about hypertension and gestational diabetes. There is *no* correlation at all, so why was that drink given to me? I bring you back to Truth #4.

A week later, at my follow-up visit, I was expecting them to give me some information about what impact this would have on me going forward, but even with my inquiry, nothing. The next visit was with a midwife, not a physician, so I was hopeful. Well, it was a disaster. They didn't even know who I was and what my history had been. I felt like I was a number, not a human, so I switched providers. I found one more local to me, but it also meant that I needed to switch hospitals. We had a hospital tour, and although it seemed fine, something was just not right.

This doctor was great. She went through my birth plan line by line with me at our first visit. She also listened to me when I wanted to wean off the (rest of) BP meds because I did not believe I was hypertensive (and had already cut the dose in half on my own). She agreed that if my MFM doctor was okay with it, she was too. I saw him the next day, and he was fine. So, I got off the meds and *never* had a high reading during the pregnancy again.

Unfortunately, the only thing she was not on the same page about was the lotus birth that I wanted. It took her a few weeks of her own research to finally come to a decision that she was not comfortable doing it. For those of you who don't know, a lotus birth is when the cord and placenta stay attached to the baby until they naturally fall off. I will get more into this in Truth #7. So, I was around 28 weeks and looking for another new provider that supported my birth plan.

While I was searching for what seemed like every practice in the three closest counties, I had taken my glucose test. You know when you are supposed to get tested for it. I was sitting in the office, drinking the super sweet drink with a large orange 100 on the bottle, thinking "wow, that's a lot of sugar." To my own ignorance, I did not realize it should have only been 50g until the results came back on my lab portal that said 50g Test, and of course, I had failed. I drank double the sugar. My results were around 150. So, I questioned the drink that I was given, but obviously, with no proof, it was she said/she said. I was instructed to take the 3-hour test and was confident that I would pass and prove the mistake. Well, clearly, the lab tech isn't super brilliant because my 3-hour results came back as follows: Fasting 146(fail), one hour 81(pass but unusual), two hour 153(fail), three hour 126 (passed). So, if you have two fails, you are labeled as a Gestational Diabetic. I had to prick my finger five times a day, every day, and monitor my sugars. So, I painstakingly did this for two weeks, I was mindful about my consumption but not super strict and I tested the limits.

When I saw my MFM doctor two weeks later, I brought my results, and he also questioned them because my logs were pretty much acceptable. I had a couple high fasting numbers, but 104 was the highest, nothing *close* to 146. He said in exact words, "Do you think they could have mixed up the vials?" Yes, validation! So, amid all this, I found the Birth Center of NJ ran by the amazing OB, Dr. Nicola Pemberton and her husband Kemonte Howard. They supported lotus birth. They accepted me despite having all these labels attached to my records. She trusted me and my ability to deliver this baby without any intervention. However, she did have hospital rights just in case of a true emergency.

For those of you keeping score, that was *two* serious misdiagnoses during this pregnancy. I fully believed that I did not have either and questioned, fought, and advocated until I was proven right. Skip ahead to Owyn's birth. He had to have his sugars tested because of the label, and he also proved that I did not have it. He was a bigger baby, so even at my 38-week MFM visit, it was questioned if I was going to have the baby delivered by 39 weeks to be safe. I told him that we would discuss it if I got the 39 weeks because I was certain I would not.

How was I certain? Because I mentioned before, this pregnancy was intuitive, and, I am a master manifester when I detach from results. Remember when I said 4/4 was the due date? Well, labor started on that day (literally the day after that conversation with my MFM doc), but I always say the Universe cannot let me have complete control when it comes to my gestations. However, I had mentioned verbally and via my social media posts two things that ring true.

☆   The last two weeks do not exist.

☆   He would be here within the next moon cycle.

Well, Owyn David was born on April 8, 2020, which was a full moon, and I was 38 weeks and 6 days pregnant. I had an unmedicated water birth without any monitors, IV, or intervention.

Are you a believer yet? You know best. You have the power. Trust yourself.

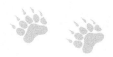

Truth 6 | YOU HAVE A RIGHT TO HAVE NON-NEGOTIABLES AND BOUNDARIES

Finances are a weight everyone carries, especially if you are about to add another human to your family. The baby industry focuses on all the stuff you need to have for this new baby. Some are true, but a lot is just fluff, and cute fluff at that. I get it. Your nesting Mama mind wants the matching bedding and all the cute nursery decor. Your family and friends shower you with clothes and blankets and all the things on your registry. But do you have anything on there for you? Do you have anything on there that supports you, nourishes you, and prepares you for the baby?

I had a support registry for my second baby. I was adamant about not having a sprinkle that Moms wanted to throw me because I did not need more stuff. I needed support. Every Mom deserves support: doulas, both birth and postpartum, a birth photographer, a lactation consultant, a date night fund, a self-care fund, and yes, some stuff, but consumable products like diapers, formula, and wipes.

I was concerned about the affordability of having a second child. However, I had non-negotiables. Doulas were part of them.

They were an investment in myself, my health, happiness, and family. Because without a happy, healthy Mama, the entire family suffers. We need to remember that as a society. Of course, the baby is a top priority, but we need to shift the care aspect to maternal health first. It's like the oxygen mask on a plane: put yours on first before your children because you cannot help them if you cannot breathe. My hope is that we also shift what is considered a luxury and what is a necessity in the birth world, and insurance is a whole other topic that I cannot even get started with. Still, the system is broken, and unfortunately, we have to build our own village.

Boundaries are so important when you are pregnant and in postpartum. It is not the time to please others. Let me say that again: it is not the time to please others. Take up space, speak up, and don't settle for anything less than what feels right. No hospital visitors. Can't hold/kiss the baby. Don't come by without calling first and asking if it's okay. Set those boundaries and stick to them. Anyone who has an issue with them needs to take a serious look in the mirror. However, most people will be respectful and empathetic towards them.

I encourage you to do this because I did not for my first, and I paid for it. Then when I spoke up, because I didn't previously put them out there, I was attacked. Mind you, the person who did the attacking is an unstable human being but set your boundaries so that it does not happen to you in the peak of postpartum. Don't put yourself in these situations. I was feeling good after my birth, and it was June, so the weather was nice. We were invited to my in-laws' for dinner. I had told my husband to make sure that their air conditioning was on because on Easter that year, it was not and it was very, very uncomfortably hot for a pregnant Mama. Their dog also needed to be locked up in their bedroom because he was screechingly loud and I did not trust him around the newborn.

Well, within minutes of us getting there, I was spun into an anxiety attack and into a massive fight with my Mother-in-law. It was about 86 degrees in the house, my feet were still swollen, and I was already sweating before Dylan was even out of his car seat. As I was taking him out, the dog showed up, screaming away. My fight or flight response never kicked in so fast than it did at that Moment. I said some words I definitely did not filter, and luckily, my husband, who was also being attacked, stood by my side, and we left.

I attribute this incident to the start of my postpartum anxiety, even though it was about five days later that the intrusive visions began. This animosity continued with Dylan for the first almost year of his life. She did not respect my boundaries and caused a lot of drama about it. Luckily, things were different with Owyn. However, it was a tough way to learn this lesson. I urge you to define and communicate your boundaries before the baby gets here. It's just as important to be on the same page as your partner, so there is no added tension that grows while you are healing.

I set strict boundaries for my second, and I was fortunate because I had COVID-19 on my side; the entire state was under quarantine the month I delivered my sweet boy, so it helped make these much easier for people to grasp. However, I laid them out as soon as I hit my second trimester, when Corona was just a beer. I gracefully explained what was and was not acceptable, and what our plans were for those initial weeks after Owyn was born.

Initially, before I decided to deliver at a birth center, we decided we would limit the number of hospital guests. With the birth center, we were discharged that same day, so there was not even an opportunity to visit. Additionally, if you were coming to visit and meet the baby, you were expected to bring a meal or help around the house in some capacity. Again, with the pandemic, not many people even tried to come over, and those who did were the closest to us, which was not even a question that they would help. They were all beyond amazing and supportive this time around, and I was able to heal and recover physically and emotionally.

Boundaries may feel uncomfortable to communicate, but you will be extremely happy you chose discomfort over a complete breakdown. Non-negotiables are your right as a woman. You are a Creator, and you deserve to define the things you feel most strongly about to make this experience the most positive one you could imagine. You are worthy of a positive pregnancy, birth, and postpartum experience. Let me repeat that; you are worthy of a positive perinatal experience.

Try This Two! What You Can Do-ula!

Take some time now and think about the experience you want to have. Not your spouse, not your Mom, not their Mom, not your best friend with three kids: you. Write down how you want to feel and how you want to sense the day of your birth and beyond. See where you need support, who can provide you that support, where you want some space or certain "rules," notice who will potentially give you an issue with them, and address any feelings that arise.

Next, define your non-negotiables. Those things you know will help create the most positive experience for you and baby (and of course, your partner too). If you'd like to go a step first and rank them by priority, so if you do need to compromise on some of them, you know which ones you feel most strongly about. Let your heart and intuition guide you on this, not your logical mind. Release all "financial obligations" from creating this list. You can figure that out later. There are ways the Universe seems to provide when you define, decide, and detach.

Lastly, write down your boundaries. Discuss them with your partner first, ensure that they are on the same page so that you are a united front if anyone questions you. Then decide the best way to communicate these boundaries to anyone who may need to hear them. The sooner, the better. Don't wait until the day before the baby is here. Review and refine this list until it feels complete and accurate.

Go to Mamabarebook.com for some journal prompts to help you get these thoughts onto paper.

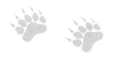

Truth 7 | YOU ARE THE MOTHER. YOU HAVE CHOICES. MAKE THEM.

Something that makes me sad about the entire perinatal experience in this country is how little the medical system thinks of women and how much information they withhold from them once becoming pregnant. Birth is uncertain to *everyone* involved, even the doctors. However, you have options on so many levels. Most women do not even know they have a choice and just go with what and when the doctor recommends. They use "safety" as a scare tactic so that you follow the path they pave for you. From the Moment you see the plus sign on the stick, you have a choice. I am not talking about that one, however. I do believe it is a woman's right to choose what is best for her wellbeing, but that topic is not what this chapter is about. In fact, it did not even dawn on me until I wrote those words.

You can choose your provider, you can choose what tests you have done, you can choose where you give birth, you can choose in what position you labor in, and you can choose what interventions are and are not acceptable. The list goes on. Birth looks different for everyone. The hostage information is where I have my gripe. Most providers don't tell you any of this. The books, the apps, the media, none of these gives insight on all the possibilities you have in front of you. *And* that *you* get to make the decision every step of the way. Of course, you can change your mind, too. You hold power to listen to your intuition and do what is best for yourself and your baby.

With Dylan, I just floated through with all the normal tests, all the protocol, and ended up at a hospital with an uneventful birth that included an IV, epidural, and some stitches. I thought I had decided on certain things, but at the Moment, I did not speak up when I noticed that no one was listening. I did not have any issues, any trauma, or any malpractice, and before I knew better, it was a great birth experience. I felt empowered by my ability to bring a human into this world. It wasn't until I crashed and burned at the hands of Postpartum Obsessive-Compulsive disorder that I threw myself into the "birth world." I focused on prevention and treatment for those Moms that also were dealing with these illnesses. But with that community, you learn much more about pregnancy, labor, birth, and beyond.

When I got pregnant with Owyn, I promised myself that I would be the one holding the steering wheel. I chose to have a lotus birth and did not stop until I found someone who supported that plan. I chose not to subscribe to the pregnancy bias that misdiagnosed me with hypertension and gestational diabetes. I chose not to be hooked up to a monitor or IV during labor. I chose to use alternative pain management methods and deliver in the water. I chose to come home hours after he was born. I chose to have a beautiful, gentle birth experience. I chose to be supported throughout it all. I chose not to circumcise, cut the cord, or have any injections given to him. I chose to breast and bottle-feed simultaneously. I chose to switch providers when I felt unheard. I chose to question the system.

Every Mother deserves to choose. In order for her to do so, she needs the information, accurately and timely. This is where I urge you to do your own research, survey other Moms, hire a doula, and question your doctor. Ask what, why, and how for anything that you do not understand, ask for alternative options or protocols. If they get defensive or unaccepting of your questions, find a new doctor. You have the choice!

I switched around 20 weeks and then again at 30 weeks, and I had an amazing experience. You are the Mother. It is your birth, baby, and life.

This doesn't stop with birth. You can choose if they watch TV or they have a tablet before they can say or spell the word "tablet." You can choose to feed them all organic purees you make yourself or buy the Gerber baby food. You can choose to keep them home or send them to school as early or later as you want. You can choose your values, beliefs, and practices that you want to instill in them. You can choose who you have them around, when, and how they should be treated.

If that is not up to your standards, return to the boundary's truth. Here's another secret. You can change your mind. You can choose one thing and then realize it is not working for your highest good, or you come into new information or an experience. You can choose to change.

Personally, Dylan had some things done, like early vaccines and circumcision, that Owyn did not have. I choose to let Dylan be a little loud and crazy in a restaurant instead of putting a screen in front of him. I chose to be truthful with him about certain things and instilled mindfulness in him as early as I could. I will do the same with Owyn. I stand my ground when I am questioned because they came out of my vagina. I get to decide what is best for them (obviously, with support from my husband).

Visit Mamabarebook.com for a complete checklist for Birth, Baby & Beyond.

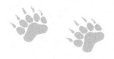
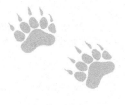

Truth 8 | LABOR IS NOT LIKE THE MOVIES

So, when I used to think of labor, what came to mind was the Hollywood version. Water breaks, rush to the hospital, scream and breathe through contractions, push, push, push, clean baby. No cord, no placenta, no days of contractions getting increasingly stronger and longer.

Now I know better.

Labor can be long. Contractions can come and go. Water can break or not. It may just leak. You have a bloody show with a teeny bit of blood or some spotting every time you go to the bathroom. You can be dilated for weeks prior to birth. You shed your mucus plug. However, all of those signs may or may not indicate that you are having a baby today. There is no clear sign: just some combination of the above, and as contractions grow stronger and longer, and you dilate more and more, then the baby is close.

There are three stages of labor. Early Labor can last hours or days. This is the time you can still keep yourself distracted and best to stay relaxed and joyful. Keep the oxytocin flowing. Active Labor is when you are in the thick of it. No turning back now. The transition is that last leg where you are about to meet the baby.

Every Mama experience labor differently. Every pregnancy can also be different. Another thing to know is that you can have back labor, which starts by feeling like bad gas pains and end up feeling like your spine is going to crack. Counter-pressure is a lifesaver for back labor. I had it with both boys.

My labor with Dylan started with what I thought was my water breaking, but it turned out it was a high leak. I had a lot of fluid with both pregnancies. It was around 3 pm Sunday when I experienced this gush and slow leak for about 30 minutes. I called my doula, got on my birth ball, and waited for contractions to start. They didn't.

Around 8 pm, I called my doctor to advise him that my water broke, and he told us to come to the hospital. Apparently, I wasn't dilated, and my fluid was still high. They had me on a monitor, and I felt some contractions, but they were light. They sent us home at around 1 am. Well, about 5 minutes after I got home, I felt these strong gas pains in my back. I thought it was just some anxiety and took a Gas X. Well, the pains were consistent and didn't go away, so around 5 am, I woke up my husband and said we were going back to the hospital. I still wasn't dilated, they kept telling me it was "false labor," I walked around the hospital floor to try to get things going. My doula was there helping me with counter-pressure. No luck. I was sent home again around 10 am Monday.

At this point, my Mom came by my house, and my doula came back as well to try to keep me comfortable. I couldn't sleep. The pain was consistent and strong. That night, I went to my Mom's for dinner, and everyone could tell how much pain I was in. That night, I labored in my glider, pushing a heating pack into my back each time they came surging. And then I would have to go to the bathroom, and some blood-tinged mucus would appear. This was a pattern all night long. That morning, I woke up, ate some peanut butter crunch cereal, and threw it up right back into the bowl. At this point, I was convinced that this was absolutely not false labor. I called my doctor and went into the office to be checked.

I was 4 cm dilated. Finally, I was going to the hospital to be admitted. They broke my water around noon. I elected to have an epidural, which took a while because getting an IV in and bloodwork from my dehydrated self was an impossible task. They finally got it after calling in the special nurse. I was on the toilet when they successfully drew it. I threw up a couple more times. The epidural was not bad to get. I just couldn't look or think about what was happening. It gave me the ability to rest for a bit. At 7:35, Dylan was born after 3 pushes, an unprepared doctor, and feeling every little bit.

That is what labor can be like.

With Owyn, I knew better, but it was still tough to not want to rush the process. My labor started at 2 am on Saturday, this time with contractions about 30 seconds long. I had been having more Braxton hicks this pregnancy, but these were more consistent. I got excited, but they tapered off a few times and came back. Then Sunday night and Monday, they were relatively gone. Tuesday morning, they started back up and were getting longer and stronger. Still no bloody show, no water leak, no other signs that he was coming.

I also had some resistance instilled in me to go "too early" to the Birth Center because I was not delivering in a hospital this time around. So, I kept my doctor in the loop, and we were taking it hour by hour. Around 10:30 Tuesday night, I did a Full Moon meditation followed by seeing some blood when I went to the bathroom. It was a teeny bit, so I was waiting for more the next time I went like with Dylan. My contractions were about 10 minutes apart, and I was able to rest for a few hours. Then around 2 am, they had me up, I went into the living room to watch a funny show, and by 4 am, I was getting to my limit. I called my doctor, crying, and she said to head up to the birth center. I arrived around 6 am, and when they checked me, I was 9cm. The midwife that was on call broke my water shortly after, and within the hour, Owyn was born.

This is what labor can be like.

My point is that it can look so different from everyone. This is where listening to your body is important and having a doula for support and education around your labor process is crucial. One thing I know for sure is labor is *not* like the movies. It is unknown to everyone, but you can stay calm, stay distracted until you can't be anymore, and stay close to your breath.

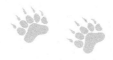
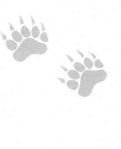

Truth 9 | BIRTH IS NOT A MEDICAL EMERGENCY

O̶ur society needs to shift our entire healthcare philosophy, but that's a separate book. This is specific to maternal care and the fact that when you add medical intervention to the birth process, that's when the statistics rise for unplanned C-sections. I say unplanned and not an emergency because there is a difference. I believe there are three types of cesareans: scheduled, unscheduled or unplanned, and a true emergency. Those that happen after induction, epidurals, and labor that "is not fast enough" for the hospital protocol are unplanned. Sometimes they are the best option for a tired Mama and a stressed baby. However, most of those situations can be avoided if the intervention did not happen.

Women should be empowered and educated about this full process, what to expect, and how to cope with the increasing surges with movement and breath. Another unknown word to most first-time pregnant Moms is oxytocin and how naturally increasing this hormone is the key to the whole process. Instead, synthetic Pitocin is injected into the system, contractions become stronger, which dominos to an epidural and then potentially, an unplanned cesarean. The birth documentary "Why Not Home?" explains this process deeply.

I love the idea of home births. It allows the process to fully manifest with comfort, support, and patience. Even though I did not have one with either of my sons, I support them. I am someone who needs to have security in place. Therefore, the increasing centers specifically for birth that are appearing more and more in this country are, in my opinion, the best option.

I had a good hospital birth with limited intervention, but I had an amazing natural birth in a tub at the birth center. The environment is different, the care is Mother centered, and the experience is looked at as natural and not an emergency.

I urge you to do some inner work, really dig deep, and shift this perception that society has ingrained in women. We do not need to fear birth. We need to embrace it. We need to be encouraged and empowered. We need to be seen, heard, and understood by the medical industry. Only then will we see a shift. Until then, you have every right to seek options for your birth. You can Manifest Your Empowered Birth. Visit Mamabarebook.com for a full self paced course to help make your ideal birth a reality.

You can still birth in a hospital with the same mindset; I am not saying that it is not the place to deliver. Just know the intention of the hospital staff and doctors is different and have a plan in place to hold true to your plan and power. Ask questions, make sure you are fully informed before making a decision that involves intervention. I know at the moment it is tough, Mama. Birth is no easy feat. That is why it is crucial to prepare and have support, whether that be your partner or a doula.

My mindset shifted so completely after Dylan's birth. I was terrified beforehand and never even knew how I could physically do it. Then I did and felt inspired. I felt so proud of myself and my body. I knew if I could do that, I could do anything. So, when I got pregnant with Owyn, it was my intention to honor that feeling and embody the power that I possessed. That is what we need to view birth as powerful and natural, not an emergency.

One last thing to mention. I recognize that there are cases that do require intervention and surgery. Safety, of course, is important to the Mother and baby. I am trying to raise awareness that it just isn't every situation and should not be the intention of the staff. Again, Mamas have a strong intuition and can recognize when that intervention is needed for the highest good of all.

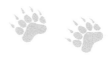
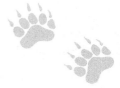

Truth 10 | YOU ARE PURE MAGIC

"There is a secret in our culture, and it is not that birth is painful but that women are strong."
Laura Stavoe

Women are the definition of miraculous, powerful beings. What we can do with our bodies is a physical phenomenon to scientists. The way our cervical tissue can stretch during labor and birth, and then contract back to its normal size is fascinating. Beyond that, the natural intelligence of the entire process of conception, gestation, and birth are astounding. We create human life with all the right cells, systems, and limbs without even consciously thinking about it, then expel it from our bodies at the exact right Moment.

We need to acknowledge this process as more than craving pickles and having swollen feet. We have to forget about what stretchmarks and cellulite will do to our appearance. We must celebrate the miracle that occurs within us each day. Pregnancy does not discriminate; you don't have to "prove you are worthy" or "good enough" to be a Creator. You innately are. Of course, there are challenges with some of us due to various factors, but speaking solely in terms of accomplishment, there is nothing that requires you to go through a test, rite of passage, or milestone before having the ability to create a life.

If that isn't magic, I do not know what is.

I am considered obese, and although other humans' perceptions of that are negative, I was able to carry, grow, and deliver two beautiful souls into this world. I am also short, have bad eyes, a slight curve in my spine, and bad posture altogether. But still, magic.

I am controlling, lazy, and impatient. I am a flawed human. All those "identifiers" are not me. I am pure magic.

As I am writing this truth, today, I was reminded by one of my mentors, "You are pure magic." And the title of this chapter has been on this page for weeks. I have never heard her say that before today. I love little universal synchronicities that validate the path I am on. I want to share this with you so that you become aware and begin to notice truly how magical you are.

I invite you to take some time and journal or meditate on these words.

I am magical.

I am a Creator.

I am enough.

I can choose what is best for me and my baby.

I am worthy of being heard.

I am supported.

I deserve to feel empowered and informed.

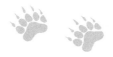

Truth 11 | YOU NEED TO PREPARE FOR WHAT COMES AFTER BIRTH TOO

We spend hours reading, researching, and seeking how to prepare for each week of pregnancy, what to expect for labor and birth, and ensuring we have all the "stuff" ready. However, we rarely worry about how to prepare ourselves for what comes after birth. Of course, no one can truly empathize with the "newborn stage" unless you have lived it, but there is a lot you can do before the baby arrives.

First, educate yourself on your options. Feeding, sleeping, burping, diapering, and bathing can look different for every Mama. Know what you want to do, but also learn other ways so you can be flexible if the baby doesn't necessarily comply. Then educate yourself on perinatal mood and anxiety disorders (PMADs) and the baby blues. You don't have to dive deep into them, but just enough to understand the symptoms so you can be aware if something arises. Being caught off guard with intrusive thoughts, rage, or inability to feel bonded with your baby can turn your world upside down if you didn't know it was possible to experience it.

Next, establish your village. Define who you will call when you need help. Notice that I didn't say, "If you need help." It truly takes a village.

That expression came to be because traditional postpartum looked different than it does today, especially in cultures in the East. Moms need time to heal and recover. They need to be nurtured and nourished while they are doing so to their babies. So, I will say it again; list who is in your village. This can be your Mom, your spouse, family, friends, or a hired specialist. Postpartum doulas are there to support your entire family during the fourth trimester. They can help with feeding support, household duties, entertaining older children, and even food preparation. If you do not have family in the area, postpartum doulas are essential.

That leads me to something else you need to prepare for before birth and do not wait until you are in the thick of sleep deprivation and giant maxi pads changes. Giving yourself grace and allowing yourself to be taken care of. Asking for what you need—lowering self-expectations. It's not forever and trust me, no one will think any less of you. You deserve this time to heal. It took about 40 weeks to create this life, so take time to recover.

Mind, body, and spirit need to adjust to your new life and the trauma that it endured. When I say trauma, I do not necessarily mean trauma in the sense of PTSD or a bad traumatic experience, but simply the physical shift your body just went through. Expansion, contraction, and all things in between. Do this inner work and give yourself permission to be what you need to be.

Lastly, decide a plan of action for yourself if you are to encounter a PMAD. Get a recommendation for a Postpartum Specialized Therapist; I cannot stress that enough. Next, decide how you feel about medication. Do you have a fear of it? If so, work through it now. Are you willing to take whatever is prescribed to you? Okay, that's fine, but also do some research on different medications so you can advocate for yourself if necessary. Then search for peer support groups either locally or virtually. These are definitely helpful when you are feeling like the only one that could possibly be going through this or having certain thoughts. Knowing you are not alone is healing. Visit Mamabarebook.com for a full self-paced program to Prepare for Postpartum. Upon completion of the course you will have a full postpartum resource guide created by you for when that time comes. In all aspects of physical, mental and spiritual health.

Try This Three: Labor Breathing

Breathe is a powerful tool that each of us possesses. It can be your anchor during labor. It brings you into the Moment and allows you to flow through the pain. Remember, each surge brings you closer to your baby, so welcome them and be grateful. Of course, as they are happening, it is tough to be in your "Zen." So, utilize these few tools to get you through each wave. Inhale for a count of 10 and exhale for a count of 10. Again, grace is needed here because it is not easy to breathe for that length of time. If you only make it to 6, 7, or 8, that is fine. You are shifting your awareness to your breath and not the pain.

Another tool is to exhale with sound or movement. Energy, specifically emotional energy, can be moved through sound. The vibrations can assist in their release. I don't know what can be more emotional than labor and birth for a woman, so this is the optimal time to use sound in addition to your breathwork.

Ask my husband how I got through the "transition" stage of labor while we were in the car driving up to the birth center, which was an hour away from our house and in the pouring rain. I was in the backseat, listening to affirmations, breathing deep, and letting out some wild sounds. No judgment or embarrassment necessary. It was exactly what I needed and can be a huge help to get through the many hours that labor can take (see Truth #8). Visit Mamabarebook.com to view a video that dives a little deeper into these practices.

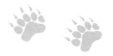

Truth 12 | BABIES NEED TO EAT, MOMS NEED TO BE HEALTHY

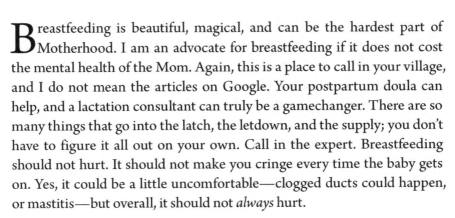

Breastfeeding is beautiful, magical, and can be the hardest part of Motherhood. I am an advocate for breastfeeding if it does not cost the mental health of the Mom. Again, this is a place to call in your village, and I do not mean the articles on Google. Your postpartum doula can help, and a lactation consultant can truly be a gamechanger. There are so many things that go into the latch, the letdown, and the supply; you don't have to figure it all out on your own. Call in the expert. Breastfeeding should not hurt. It should not make you cringe every time the baby gets on. Yes, it could be a little uncomfortable—clogged ducts could happen, or mastitis—but overall, it should not *always* hurt.

If your nipples crack and bleed and come out a different shape than they went in, have them looked at. The baby could have a tie of some sort or the baby's position may need to be adjusted. There are butters to help your nipples and there are devices that can help this, too, but they are temporary fixes. It's important to be evaluated by a lactation specialist. I am not an expert. Just a Mom who stopped breastfeeding with Dylan quickly because I didn't know better.

With Owyn, I am now three months into nursing him. Not exclusively, but on our own terms. It does not have to be all or nothing. There are safe medications you can be on and breastfeed. You do not have to choose between feeding your baby and your mental health. You can decide what feels right for you. Go with that.

If your baby has an allergy or an intolerance, you may need to supplement. If your supply is not there, do not feel inadequate. You are allowed to make the best decision for you and your baby when it comes to feeding. The fact is they need to eat, and they need a healthy Mom. If breastfeeding does not serve you, let it go. Try as much as you need to to feel good about letting it go.

Again, I nurse Owyn a couple of times a day. We have a beautiful bond, he gets nutrients and antibodies needed from them, and I feel empowered by being able to nurse him with my body. I tried to exclusively breastfeed with him. My supply was not there, and he lost a lot of weight in the first week. I also had bleeding nipples within the first two days. I ordered nipple shields, which helped with that, but it was such a task to feed him with them. Then I decided to exclusively pump, so he was still getting the milk but just not from my breast directly. I wasn't pumping enough to keep up with him, and I missed actually having that bonding with him on me. So, I found my "right fit."

He is formula-fed so that he receives enough milk, is gaining adequate weight, and is healthy but we also get to bond, and I can provide him nutrients and antibodies from my source. To summarize, breastfeeding is personal to every Mother. The best advice I can give is that it does not have to be all or nothing, keep your own mental health in mind, there are support and aids to help you in your journey, and you are enough, no matter what.

Truth 13 | THIS SH*T IS HARD

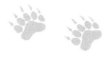
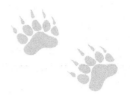

Stop comparing yourself to the highlight reel. There is nothing real about it. No Mother has it all together. No Mother has all the answers. Motherhood is tough. Creating the life inside you for 9 months is technically the easy part if we are speaking in relative terms.

You are enough for your baby. You are exactly what he or she needs. Stop looking at the InstaMoms that only post the precious Moments. Motherhood is raw. Motherhood is messy. Motherhood is magical. It's so many things at any given Moment. We all experience it differently, but it is not easy.

Sure, it can be easier for some to adapt to the change and some babies may be easier than others, but it is not easy. I have said it a few times already, but it is worth saying again; give yourself grace. You do not have to be perfect. You can make mistakes, and trust me, you will. You can get frustrated, upset, and overwhelmed. You can cry your ugliest cry. Just remember to celebrate all the little victories as well. Remember to be grateful for all the things you are. Remind yourself how powerful and strong you are. You grew that little baby, birthed them Earthside, and now you have such unconditional love for this tiny soul so you can also have that same love for yourself because they are a part of you, an extension of your soul.

Sleep deprivation, hormonal fluctuations, and constant neediness can wear on anyone. The first three months are a warzone, but trust me, you will make it through. Know it is temporary. It gets better; it gets easier. You gain confidence along the way. You are doing the best you can with what you have at every Moment. If something feels beyond your ability to cope, please seek help. You are not alone, it is not your fault, there is help for you, and you will be well once again.

Not to mention, you are doing all of this while bleeding. It seems like the 9 months of cycles you missed come whirling back all at once, and you experience the longest period ever. Some women even experience uterine contractions a few days after birth, especially if they are breast-feeding. I don't remember experiencing them with Dylan, but I for sure did with Owyn, and boy, it was tough. Bleeding, feeling your back spasm while you are trying to feed your newborn and soak up all the goodness is hard. But take it day by day, Moment by Moment. If you aren't sure if a clot or feeling is common or normal, please reach out.

Your body, no matter how beautiful and gentle your birth was, went through trauma. It needs time to heal. The standard in this country is 6 weeks, but truly, it takes months and maybe even longer to fully recover. Honor that time. Don't give yourself so many expectations to bounce back. You will never be the woman you were before. You will never go back. You are already more powerful, stronger, and more evolved than ever before. So, if you lose the baby weight and regain your muscle tone, celebrate it in a different way. Not as bouncing back, but as propelling yourself forward.

Additionally, there is no need to rush this process or even feel pressured to take steps to do it. You are perfect the way you are, and when you feel good, you will do good. So, focus on that. Focus on feeling good and enjoying these Moments, because they go fast. Focus on tuning into your body and listening to what it is telling you. Rest when you need to rest, move when you need to move, and find stillness when you need silence.

Society has been under such duress in the last couple thousand years, we have lost our way in terms of honoring feminine energy and the divine feminine gifts that we all possess. We have been conditioned to hustle, strive, and climb for power, wealth, and control. This model doesn't allow for women to heal and recover after birth; it promotes a race to get back to normalcy. However, it is not realistic, and we need to dissolve this notion as much as we possibly can. We must look within and follow what we know we need, rather than trying to prove yourself to the patriarchy.

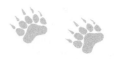
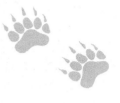

Truth 14 | MARRIAGES NEED TLC TOO

Here's some more real talk: marriage is hard. Marriage with a new baby or two can be catastrophic. As I am writing this, I just huffed and puffed at my husband for insisting that I take the baby up with me to write some chapters, because I have been behind on my deadline, was home with both boys all day, and just wanted to have a few minutes of peace to write and feel productive since my doula is here. I only have her for two more weeks. Why doesn't he get it? Why does he get to sleep? Why doesn't his body morph and stretch? Why isn't his natural reaction to cry and worry?

There is a lot of frustration and resentment that can erupt when you are pregnant and postpartum. There are a lot of expectations and sometimes by no fault of their own, a lack of empathy for you, because how on Earth could any man understand what we as women go through during this whole perinatal journey? Sometimes the strongest-looking marriages can implode for reasons un-be-knownst to the world, i.e., Rachel and Dave Hollis' that was just announced and crushed me.

Well, my husband and I have been married for just about eight years, and we said "I do" just three months after we met (enter gasp here). However, we have been through some adversity together. A cross-country move and move back, illness and death in our close families, dog surgery, fertility treatments, each had our fair share of mental health issues, two pregnancies, two births, two houses, very different families and upbringings, and sometimes completely opposite views on life. Sometimes I worry about how we are ever going to make it, after being a child of divorce and knowing so much of it.

However, I feel like we always come back to neutral, to our true north. We share one solid foundation. We both have a high concern for the other's happiness, as well as our own. We make sacrifices for each other, but we also fill our own cups first, then we enjoy the goodness that fills them together and allows it to pour over onto our boys.

I am not saying it is easy. I am just saying that I have a lot of hope that even though we disagree on a lot and may not see the world the same way, we care about each other, and we have a passion for each other that keeps us going. It takes work, it takes communication (which is not always easy), and it takes love. It takes compromise and empathy, even though it's not always possible. It takes compassion and will, *and when there is a will, there's a way.*

I remember distinctly hearing a radio interview or a reference to an interview on the radio while driving to work one morning a couple of years ago, how Kelly Rowland said she puts her husband before her children and is getting some "beef" about it. But she stated how the relationship and love created those children, and it was important to prioritize that as much as it is to prioritize our children. That stuck with me. Even if I am exhausted, I try to make him happy or put in a little extra effort, and he does the same.

Marriage is like a newborn. It needs to be fed, rested, and kept clean. Do your best each day to unconditionally love that other person (if he/she is not emotionally or physically abusive). Take interest in each other, check in with them, see what you do that annoys the crap out of them, and try to work on it. Trust me, there are things.

Keep two things in mind when in the bedroom (or car, couch, or shower; parents must get clever).

1. If he was in the delivery room, he has some concept of what happened, so he knows that your body may not be perfect. You criticize yourself more than he ever will, so feel good and sexy

about yourself. Let him compliment you. Let him touch you. And let him pleasure you (of course, only consensually).

2. Speak up. Tell him what you want, how you want it, if it hurts, or it feels strange. He cannot read your mind. You just had your body expand and contract in the areas he now wants to play with. They may feel different. He will not know that you need to tell him, lovingly and proactively. I will be transparent here. My husband and I have a great sex life. It has gotten better and better over the years. We have tried new things, and I know what I like, when I like it, how I want it, and he listens. I do the same in return. Sometimes I am tired and reluctant to do anything, but afterward, I am usually the one reaping the benefits.

Mamas, please be comfortable with yourself. Be comfortable with your orgasms. Believe you are worthy of them each time. I say them because you can have more than one. If you do not know how, or you don't find sex enjoyable, explore and play with yourself first. You cannot expect your partner to do something you cannot even do for yourself. If there are issues in this area, please seek a counselor or specialized therapist. You deserve to have a healthy sexual relationship, just like a healthy physical and emotional one.

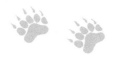

Truth 15 | YOUR BABIES ARE TRULY WISE. TAKE NOTICE.

As parents, we have the right and responsibility to raise good humans. However, in my experience, that phrase should be changed to "we have the right and responsibility to preserve the goodness in them." Babies have a natural intelligence that we cannot even understand as adults. That part of us was lost by our societal and generational conditioning. They have the concept of love, equality, and freedom from the Moment they are born. They live completely in the present and do not judge, blame, or doubt themselves. They feel all their emotions as they happen. They communicate when their needs must be met. They are completely accepting of who they are, what they look like, and see the world exactly as it is, not what they perceive it to be.

Our babies feel the energy. They rely on all their senses for the better part of the first year and beyond. They absorb so much knowledge and grow so much within such a short period of time. They don't see color, gender, sexual orientation, religion, socioeconomic status, or any other label that we have been conditioned to give ourselves. You can put any baby next to each other, and they will all react purely based on senses, instinct, and love.

I was fortunate to learn Reiki prior to having my children. I am also grateful that I went through the darkness with Dylan because it forced me to rely on my meditation practice. He felt my energy. Of course, he did, so when it was time for him to sleep, I could not be the anxious mess I was. I invested in my favorite meditation experiences, and we listened to it every single night while he fell asleep on my chest. Now he is three, and we still listen to them each night I put him to sleep.

I have been fortunate to have two babies that have been great sleepers, and considering the horror stories I heard about my own sleep habits as an infant, I can only attribute this to the peacefulness and energy work that I do with both as they head into their slumbers. They do not judge the life force. They do not have preconceived notions or skepticism about it like most adults that I encounter do. They just accept and receive it. They allow it to heal and restore them. They are wise beyond their years.

As Mothers, I feel we put the weight of the world on our shoulders to make sure we are teaching our children all the "right stuff." How to eat organically. How to succeed in school and the world. How to be social, share, be respectful, and how to (fill in just about anything here). If we just observed and interfered less, we may have a better chance of preserving this innate goodness.

Try This Four: Learn from your littles

Observe. Watch and listen as they go through their day. See life through their eyes. Journal on all the wisdom you find. Notice their presence, their emotions, and their communication. Then compare it to that of you, a conscious-minded adult that adds narratives, judgments, and internal stories to everything by no fault of your own. It is how we have all been conditioned. But when we know better, we can do better. So, do this for a day. If that feels too heavy, then just do it for an hour. See what you can learn from them. Then see if you can implement those learnings. Notice how your world begins to shift. Notice how they begin to elevate their vibrations as well as yours.

Create this cycle of learning so that you are in checks and balances. Of course, as parents, we have a responsibility to teach our children the ways of the world. However, I fully and completely feel that we have an equal responsibility to learn from them so we can reflect it back in the most appropriate way. We need to preserve and cherish those innate qualities we are all born with and somehow fade away from. Just make a commitment to try this for one hour, one day, one week, and see how your life changes.

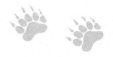

Truth 16 | YOUR STORY CAN SAVE

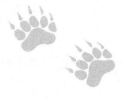

Do you know how many Moms struggle in the newborn phase? Do you know how many of those Moms continue to struggle for months or maybe even years after their babies are born? If you have encountered adversity, anxiety, depression, rage, intrusive thoughts, or anything during your experience as a Mother, I beg of you, speak up. Do not hide it. Do not be ashamed of those thoughts, feelings, or emotions.

You are not alone. You are part of the majority. We can change the narrative if we share our stories, no matter how awful they seem to us. The struggles to bond with your baby, the thoughts of harm, the constant worries, the feelings of grief, and overwhelm. They are all common.

Your body, mind, and spirit just went through an expansiveness over the last 10 months to produce another human that needs you constantly to care for it as you recover from trauma yourself, all without the sleep needed to function as your hormones try to regulate themselves back before gestation. You think that all Moms are having a super easy time and you are the only one feeling this way? Nope! When I first had my visions with Dylan, it threw me straight into 24/7 anxiety.

I spoke up the minute it happened. I screamed for help and for them to stop. I sought support from my Mom, my doulas, my OB, the therapist he recommended, and my entire village. Even with immediately speaking up and having the support of all those people, I was in complete darkness for weeks. I couldn't find the worth in all of it. I knew I loved my baby more than anything in this world, but why was I attacking my own mind? Why were these thoughts, visions, and feelings taking over?

Why couldn't I stop them? They must have been true if I could not control them.

I was terrified of snapping one day and acting on them. I was terrified that I wouldn't be here anymore. I was terrified life was going to get the best of me. Everything triggered me: household objects, rooms and structures, news headlines, social media posts, commercials, and TV shows. I unfollowed 800 people on Facebook and then deactivated it. I only watched Bravo TV because they only showed their own shows as commercials. The Real Housewives and Million Dollar Listing NY became all I knew.

As I sat with Dylan, I fed him, watched him sleep, and tried to just make it through. My therapist definitely helped. She validated my feelings, educated me on risk factors and why it made sense I was experiencing these things. She educated me on the spectrum of disorders, and why it was X and not Y, and helped me understand the medications available so that I was no longer afraid of them.

Once I stopped resisting the medication, I began to feel better. It was able to get me to a neutral place and then begin to build myself back up to the Mom I wanted to be. About 18 months after Dylan was born, I shared my story publicly in detail. Since then, I have not stopped sharing. I tell it any chance I get so that other Moms know what can happen and how to prepare for it if it does. Also, so that they know they are not alone, and there are hope and support. There are so many resources out there for new Moms; you just must know where to look. Unfortunately, your OB/GYN usually is not that place.

Here is the original version of my story that I first shared publicly and truly began to heal and started the path to help others:

But this does not define you. This is not who you are.
You know who. You. Are.

Moana

That song, I have heard about 100 times since October (It was February when I wrote this), and no, not an exaggeration. For anyone who has a toddler, you understand.

But not until I had my latest anxiety episode did it truly resonate with me and who I am.

So, I am sharing my PMAD story, for the first time in this much detail, because I can finally open up holistically about the thought, emotions, and actions that occurred in those months following birth.

It all started on a Friday Night.

Up until that Moment, I had felt empowered as a Mom. I was dealing with recovery fine, I was proud of my "northern lights" as I called my new stretch marks because of the way they formed sideways, and although breastfeeding was a bit painful, I was okay with supplementing formula due to Dylan's jaundice.

I even passed the PPD test my Doulas had given me just days before. Other than the incident with an inconsiderate nameless person that threw me into a tizzy a mere four days after having my beautiful son, I was doing just fine.

And then John ran to pick up Chinese food. Dylan was in his pack and play. And thoughts of knives and him flashed before me. I instantly was anxiety-ridden. I called my Mom, who came by and walked with me 'til I was calm, but the emotion just poured out. She called my doulas for advice. But again, it was Friday night, so nothing anyone could truly do until Monday morning.

So that weekend, I was anxious, anticipating Monday thinking, "okay I just have to get to Monday." I was a mess. The thoughts kept creeping in, Dylan in the washing machine, Dylan in the bathtub, just any possible scenario he could get hurt in the house.

I went to the doctor's Monday, he prescribed Xanax and Zoloft and gave me a recommendation for a therapist.

I filled the Xanax but not the Zoloft I barely took them but felt better just having them.

I scheduled an appointment with the therapist and just had to wait until I met with her to feel safe.

I was waiting for someone to validate that I wasn't going to snap. That I wasn't going to lose it. I had no idea why these thoughts were happening, but I knew I was terrified.

For the next few weeks, I was in an anxious state almost constantly. I refused to be alone with the baby or by myself, so every morning, I would wake up, pack a bag, and head to my Mom's house as John left for work. My sister was home too with my niece, who is 3 weeks older than Dylan.

I would stay there until John got home then head back. This repeated every day. I could not even be alone downstairs too long. John could not even go out to his car to grab something without me freaking out. I just thought "it" whatever this madness was, was waiting for the one chance or Moment for me to "snap." Like it was something out of my control and external from me.

I then started getting visions of hurting myself. I was triggered by Chester Bennington's tragic loss. It scared me to the core because he was such a positive person in interviews, and the song he had released with Kiera that I liked a lot then seemed like a warning sign to the world that no one picked up on. So needless to say, my disorder took this information and ran with it. I had visions of hurting myself, hanging from rafters, taking too many pills, and just awful images filled my brain.

Then there were talks of nuclear testing and North Korea, so thoughts spiraled of all impending doom and why are we even here, this world scares the shit out of me. I was seriously at a breaking point. And just a reminder I had a newborn who needed my love, care, and sane mind.

I only could only watch shows that were upbeat or mindless. I couldn't see, hear, or talk about any news or headlines and would stop anyone who brought up anything that I couldn't handle.

I couldn't hear the word suicide, and I couldn't have a knife at my place setting or even on the table.

It was completely overtaking my life.

During this time, I went to therapy. I did meditate and self- healed, but it only helped at the Moment.

So finally, I made the decision to go on the medication I was prescribed.

And guess what! It helped. I elongated my suffering a good three weeks because I was stubborn, embarrassed, and ashamed that I couldn't beat this on my own.

It did take a few weeks to kick in fully, I slowly began feeling normal again, in control of my life. Not ridden with anxiety and fright.

I was able to go out in public without thinking the worst would happen. I was able to socialize without someone saying something that would trigger me.

I was still cautious. But everything got better as time passed. I still, to this day, have certain uncomfortableness with that word and again cannot watch any violent TV even like SVU.

Postpartum OCD changed me, that is for certain. But it does not get to define me as a Mother or the Woman I am for the rest of my life.

I am still on the medication because it allows me to live empowered and be the person I am.

I am finally able to share, and beyond that, I want to help others and spread proactive awareness about postpartum mood disorders (PPMD). Maybe this story would have been a little different if I would have known that PPOCD existed, and I was a perfect candidate for it to happen.

I am so thankful for those in my family and the caring doctors, therapists, and doulas that helped me through this darkness. But now I am on a mission to be another Mama's light.

Thank you for reading this to the end. Dylan is almost 2. I am finally able to create my definition of life.

I cannot explain to you how healing it was to divulge my truth. Other Moms began to reach out and share their own struggles with me because they did not feel alone. I encourage you to share your challenges, triumphs, good days, bad days, and do not be ashamed of anything you encounter in Motherhood, because your story can save others.

Truth 17 | "THIS" DOES NOT DEFINE YOU

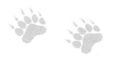

During much of Dylan's first year of life, I was rebuilding myself after what I can only describe as the scariest time of my life. Around 5 to 6 months is when I made the decision that this illness was not going to define me as a Mother. I began working on myself, holding myself accountable to him, in terms of making sure my cup was full. I stayed true to my mindfulness practices, began learning more, evolving more, and helping more. I had purpose and intentions, I built a community, and have since been on a continuous journey to keep going, to keep forging onward to help other Moms and helping myself.

I decided that my postpartum story was not my identifier. I decided that I was going to define my Motherhood. I decided that I was going to make myself a priority for my family's sake. Every single day, I make a choice to be my best self. Some days that means binging Netflix and cuddling with my boys. Other days, it means transforming lives with the gifts I have found along the way.

The point is, I make the choice, give myself grace when I need to, and I define the kind of Mother I am, not society, my parents, or my ego. I offer you this suggestion; never stop defining who you are. Set intentions for yourself and take steps each day to be that person. Sometimes you will fall short and on others, you will climb mountains.

Don't allow any illness, highlight reel, self-judgment, past trauma, or unworthiness win. You are divine. You are a Creator. You make the decision. My life has not been the same since I made the decision back when Dylan was 6 months old. I am living in cause. I choose the effects.

Motherhood can be the greatest time of your life. It reveals your strengths, your fullest heart, and all the beautiful energies of this world. It brings you back to your playful nature. You find the simplest things to celebrate. You laugh at the cutest sounds. You are instantly melted by the most enamoring phrase that comes out of their mouth, and you just can't believe that you just heard what you heard.

This is the life you get to be part of. The challenges, struggles, and hard days just even it out. We live in polarity. If you honor that, you can lean into both without judgment and self-criticism. Again, you get to define who you are as a Mother and all the other identities you take on in your life. Sit with this a bit. Take time to visualize your best self. Remember to be grateful for everything that has led you to this Moment—reading this Truth, in this book, on this day. You are magic.

You can evolve. Once you feel like you found yourself, dig deeper. Life continues to reveal new guideposts to you. I first began this journey with my focus as mindful parenting, then realized the power was in my story and drifted towards Mamas who were also experiencing postpartum mood and anxiety disorders (PMADs). I was able to show them there was a transformation that happened as time went on. Finally, after having Owyn, I realized that there was a crucial need to lift up women throughout the entire perinatal journey, which is where I am today. With my experiences, training, certifications, and constant self-investment, I can define my life, my purpose, and my role as a Mother in each Moment.

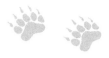
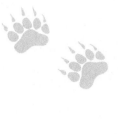

Truth 18 | YOU WILL SURVIVE TODDLERDOM

Toddlers. Need I say more? I guess so, since I am writing a book and that is kind of the whole point. I always thought that the newborn phase was the hardest, especially considering my experience with Dylan. Now, after having Owyn, the newborn phase can be magical, if you are not knee-deep in darkness and intrusive thoughts. Infants are adorable, and as they learn to eat foods, walk, and talk, they step into their little selves.

Then it hits. Toddlerdom. I know you have heard the terms "terrible twos" and "threenagers." Well, it can be true. Not because they are terrible or attitude-y, but because they are learning emotions. They are living fully in those emotions and expressing them as they occur. It's called emotional intelligence. However, generational conditioning has led most of our parents to teach toddlers to "calm down," "stop crying," "behave," etc. Especially boys. There is a tragic suppression of any emotion that may be considered "weak" for little boys. The phrases like "man up" or "toughen up" really get to me.

We need to encourage our toddlers to *feel* the emotions, be able to communicate them, process them, and permit them to explore them. That will only benefit them later on. Of course, we still need to teach them to behave in aspects of violence, respect, and boundaries but let them experience all the big emotions how they need to. Let them cry, hold space when they tantrum, and tell them it is okay and that they are safe and loved.

It is heart-wrenching to go through as a Mom, but it is inevitable. Also, give yourself a lot of grace. You will get frustrated with them. You will yell and say the wrong thing. You are only human. Forgive yourself and try to do it differently next time.

Also, as parents, it is crucial to be on the same page about this. Make sure it is something you discuss and have a plan, regardless of what that may be for your family on how you handle this phase. Whether you are a gentle parent, believe in time out, or a light spanking, I am not here to judge and dictate what is right. All I am trying to say is that both parents need to be on equal wavelengths. This allows the toddler to understand the boundaries and what is and isn't acceptable behavior. They will push those limits every single day. They are learning.

One thing to remember is they are basically a subconscious mind at this point in time. They need clear direction and limited use of words that contradict what you are saying. Don't, stop, and no are negative tenses and the subconscious mind only here's what comes next. For example, if I say "Don't think of blue dogs." What are you thinking of? Remember that next time you tell a toddler "Don't scream, jump or hit" and find them doing exactly the opposite.

You need to be consistent for everyone's sake. Again, it will probably not come naturally to you, but if you are mindful, it can be achieved. If you truly consider all the toddler is learning during these years, how could they not be filled with emotions and rebellious tendencies?

Like all phases of Motherhood, it is temporary; you will get through. Just breathe.

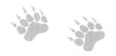

Truth 19 | Transition to Two Can Be Easier Than You Think

I was the typical Mama, so scared to bring a second baby into our family. What if Dylan doesn't take well to him? What if I can't handle both of them? How could I possibly love the second as much as the first? I felt guilty to make Dylan have to share my attention. I felt scared that it would be the same experience as the first time.

I felt so many emotions. I kept procrastinating when we were going to start trying. The idea was there, but the execution was not until I got that beautiful surprise (see Truth #2). Even when we got that positive result, the emotions and anxieties fluttered all throughout my pregnancy. How on Earth was this going to play out? The baby did not even have a room since we were hosting an exchange student who was going to be here until after his due date. So, there was no nursery decorating, no baby shower (not that I wanted one), and all the hand-me-downs from Dylan. We were not prepared financially, either.

But guess what? It all worked out. That is the message here, Mama. You do not need to drive yourself crazy with all the guilt, questioning yourself, and anxiety about *how*. It just works out. I can say this with confidence because my birth and postpartum happened in a global pandemic, when the world was upside down, and we faced unprecedented phenomena throughout it all. Somehow—financially, emotionally, physically—it just all worked out.

There will be challenges, of course. Dylan is a typical hyper 3-year-old who doesn't understand his own strength and energy. He loves tugging, pulling, and pressing on every inch of the baby. It is quite terrifying, but we are all surviving. It comes from a place of affection and love, which is the most important. We only went through a week or so of "I don't like baby Owyn," and "Put him down." It did not last, and he is such a proud big brother. We make sure that he has his own time with each of us, and he understands that he has certain things that the baby cannot have and vice versa.

I was also fortunate in the potty-training era. Dylan's first day without a diaper was on Christmas Eve last year (2019). Owyn was born on 4/8/2020. He never regressed or wanted anything to do with diapers, even though he saw Owyn in them. However, he likes to be up close and personal when we change a poopy one though (oh, boys!). About 9 or 10 weeks after Owyn was born, Dylan stopped wearing one overnight as well. I was warned that potty training the oldest too close to the birth can have some repercussions, but there were not any with us, so go with your gut on this one, Mama. If you feel they are ready, forge ahead. Also, if you have a little boy, here is the best advice I can give you. Ready for it?

When potty training a boy, sit them backward on the toilet. No splash concerns, they can watch it come out so they can get the concept quicker, and also, the way the toilet is structured, they actually sit by the narrow part, so they do not fall in. Now Dylan is tall enough to scooch himself up on the toilet and go all by himself. He calls me in if I need to wipe him, but otherwise, he is self-sufficient. It's awesome!

Grace is super important during literally all of Motherhood but worth mentioning here. You need to know that it's going to be chaotic. It is going to be messy, but most of all, it is going to be beautiful. If you are reading this book before you have your first baby or any baby after that, you are now prepared and informed so you can go into it knowing ways to prevent PMADs from taking over, just how important your village is, and how extremely powerful you are.

Transition to two ain't got nothing on you!

Try This Five: Breathing with Your Baby

Smell the _____ (cookies, flowers, candy, popcorn). Anything that smells strongly to trigger a big inhale. Now, blow the _____ (bubbles, candles, worries) away. Anything that lets out a big exhale. When they seem overwhelmed or overly living in emotions, teach them to come back to their breath in this fun and easily understood way.

Spoiler alert: It helps you, as the parent, do the same thing. If you get into this habit when they are in a neutral state or as a routine, it can be easily used when they get hyped up. Don't try it only in tantrum mode. It will not work. It has to be a learned response before it can be implemented. If you want to dive even further, you can meditate with your baby, do yoga, chant, or do some tapping. All these tools can help them over the course of their lives in the sense of coping with stress, emotions, and health. Tapping is an amazing tool to utilize. All you need is your hands. If you go to Mamabarebook.com, you will be able to find a few videos that are geared for both Mothers and little ones.

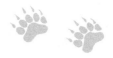
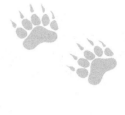

Truth 20 | YOU CAN PARENT ON PURPOSE

Most of the time, we, as humans, are set to autopilot, especially once we become sleep deprived. Busy parents are just trying to stay afloat with schedules, responsibilities, and livelihood. However, you can make a conscious choice to parent on purpose. What am I talking about? I am giving you permission to parent the way you want to. The way you see fit. The way that feels best for you, not what you have been conditioned to believe you are supposed to do.

Vaccinate or not. Homeschool or not. Let your kids run around naked all over the house or not. It is up to you. Do what you believe is best while you are pregnant, for your birth, and especially with your babies. I am sure you love and respect your parents, grandparents, in-laws, and everyone else in your family and the mainstream media. But for goodness sake, you can do what you want without any guilt. Stand firm and go with your gut.

Our generation is unlike any other before us. We are awakening. We are innovative. We are purposeful. Empathy runs deep, and connection is more important than ever. So, when you choose to do something that seems out of the realm of normalcy, push on. No matter what adversity or controversy that may arise. Simply acknowledge their suggestion, thank them for their intention, and do whatever you freaking want.

You birthed those babies. You will raise them to be good humans. I have faith in you. With that being said, you cannot do this if you do not choose to parent on purpose. I am not saying you must be "on" all the time but be mindful when it seems like you are coasting along. Implement routines in your day with your family. Implement time for work, play, and purpose. Believe you are worthy of making your family the best it can be, whatever that looks like.

I began meditating with Dylan since he was born. Now you are probably asking, how can a newborn can meditate? They technically cannot. However, I began a routine. We listened to meditation while he had his last bottle of the night as he drifted to sleep. I did some reiki and then put him down. He was sleeping from 8 pm to 6 am by 3 months. I only credit that to the Reiki and stillness.

I have not been able to do the same with Owyn, and he is approaching 3 months, and although he is a good sleeper, he is not to that level. I also began using singing bowls, yoga, gratitude boards, and crystals throughout the last three years. Dylan immediately takes to all things mindful and "woo woo." He is my moon child. He even chants Sanskrit Mantras like *Om Shanti Om* with me and lights up from it.

Owyn has the energy-baby quality that Dylan had as well. I still Reiki him each day but just not in the nightly way I did with Dylan. I cannot wait to see how he blossoms with these practices as well.

You do not have to do all these things to parent on purpose. I am just sharing those things that I chose to do with them. Yours can look vastly different. The important thing is the intention behind it. Make that clear and use action steps to create habits. It doesn't have to be a perfect formula. It can be mismatched and patchy, but whenever you can be, be.

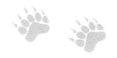

Truth 21 | YOU CREATE LIFE. YOU CAN CREATE THE LIFE YOU WANT.

Motherhood has taught me a strength I never knew I had. As women, we possess this innate power within us all to create. We are alchemists. We alchemize food into waste, eggs and sperm into babies, and all our energy into our realities. No matter what you believe, universal laws and quantum physics prove certain truths. We are energy. Everything is energy.

There is a natural intelligence within us that grows, nourishes, and essentially builds a human using only our bodies without any conscious or logical effort. I may have mentioned this throughout the book, but honestly, it's something I wish that women can be reminded of every day of their lives. We are so minimized, patronized, and almost ostracized in this society that pregnancy is seen as weakness and birth as a medical emergency.

Let me remind you again. You create a life with your body without consciously waking up and deciding to make a foot or a lung. So, you're telling me that you cannot create anything you desire in this world?

I am here to remind, encourage, inspire, and empower you to step fully into who you are. Love yourself completely and deeply. Accept all that is within. Know what you are capable of. And drown out the societal and generational crap that you have been fed your entire existence.

You can decide what kind of Mother you are. You have the opportunity and ability to raise good humans in this crazy world. You have all you need to change any circumstance that comes forth. You are as magical as your baby's smile.

I am proof that you can create the life you want. Even during a pandemic, we are flourishing. I am so blessed, and some may say it is a coincidence. But I believe it is intention, vibration, and decision. I continuously invest in myself, learn new ways to help others, and serve those who need me. I fill my cup so I can overpour to those I love. As Moms, we need to put ourselves first. For the sake of our families, we need to be healthy, happy, and certain in our power.

If your current situation is not serving your highest good, then it is your responsibility to change it. Create a new situation. Create a new reality. All of life is an illusion. It is your perception of this world. You can create abundance, love, wealth, luck, vibrancy, community, and service. You have a purpose.

My intention for this book is to give you a gleam of hope that Mamas are the most badass beings on the planet and motivate you to effect change in your own life, whether or not you have taken the rite of passage from woman to Mother. From conception to Mothering adult children, it is no easy feat. However, I could not imagine this world without the power, strength, and love of a Mom.

You are important. You are worthy. You are a Creator. No matter what life seems to throw at you, remember that you have the power to create the life you want.

I hope, in some way, you have been inspired, motivated, or enraged to go within and find the power and light that you hold. We are miracle makers. You, yourself, are also a miracle. Go ahead, bring your hands up to your heart. Feel it beating. That is miraculous.

Your body works so hard for you without your ego mind interfering. Understand that same concept when creating, carrying, and birthing a child. Then, apply that concept to anything else in your life. Have the faith and belief that you can create the life that you desire in every aspect, just how you have faith and belief that you will wake up tomorrow or that water is wet.

You get to choose. You get to decide. And most importantly, you get to create. Thank you, beautiful Creator. Thank you.

Gratitude for You

I am profoundly grateful for you. See, we are all connected, and taking this time to read these pages contributes to the collective consciousness of the world. It moves us toward changing the narrative around women and conception, women and pregnancy, women and Motherhood, women and power. I urge you to take this information, share it, scream it, and create your own experiences. Share your stories, make your decisions, and feel the magic within. Lean into those little joyful Moments, learn from your babies, and take notice of your world through their eyes. I want to know your triumphs, challenges, aha-Moments, and all the things you have gone through in your maternal journey.

Go to **Mamabarebook.com** to connect and share your story.

Remember, it can save!

From my heart to yours, thank you!

Made in the USA
Columbia, SC
08 October 2020

22383605R00049